KALEA & HER

Sweet Tooth

SUGAR MUSEUM
IN SWEETNESS WE TRUST

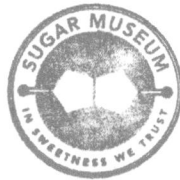

BY TERRI HUGHES-OELRICH

Sugar Museum, San Diego
info@sugarmuseum.org
www.sugarmuseum.org

Please contact Terri Hughes-Oelrich at thugheso@sdccd.edu
or the Sugar Museum at info@sugarmuseum.org.

Written and illustrated by Terri Hughes-Oelrich.

Interior layout and cover design by Monica Hui Hekman of
MH Art & Design

Edited by Debbie Millikan, Yvette Dibos, Tom Andrew,
Theresa Copley and many others.

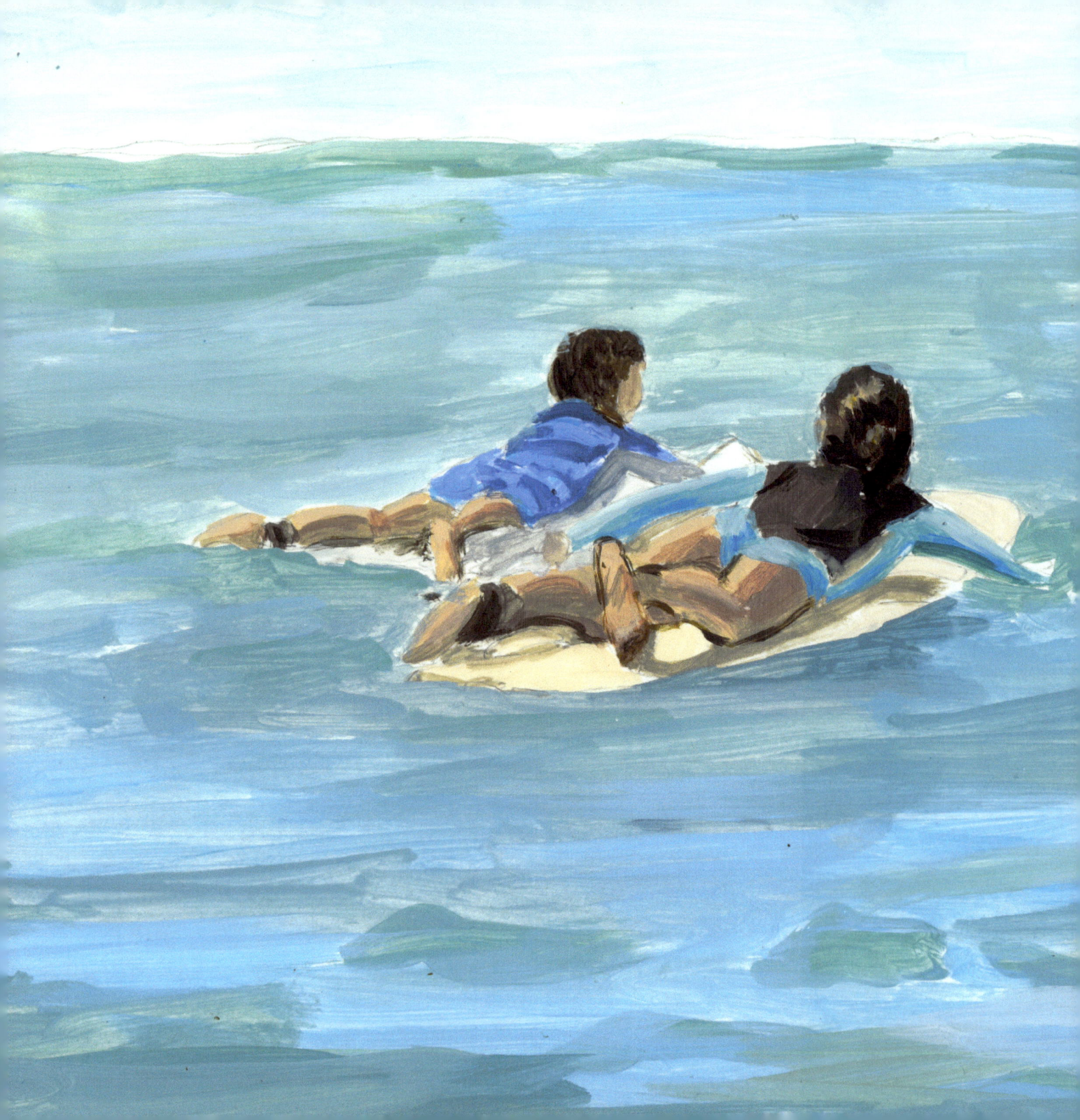

One Morning

Kalea and her mom were paddling out into the surf near Diamond Head, Hawaii. She began to dream about donuts, powdery and warm. "Hey Mom, when was the last time we went to that donut shop after surfing?" Her mom was quiet, pondering her childhood and stopping for donuts on the way home from surfing with her dad.

Kalea often dreamed about her favorite sweets; crepes with cherries and whipped cream, chocolate layer cake, lemon bars, ... Her sister McKenzie paddled up to her and said, "Hey Kalea, I bet you can't go a whole day without sugar."

"What?" she yelled back, "I don't need sugar, I can go a whole week!"

Her mom just smiled.

Day One

As Kalea got the salt water out of her hair, she smelled french toast and hurried to the breakfast table.

"Mom, does this have sugar in it?"

Her mom put some lemon in her tea and said, "Kalea, you know how to read the labels. Look at the ingredients!"

So Kalea read the labels on the bread, eggs and milk. She was safe.

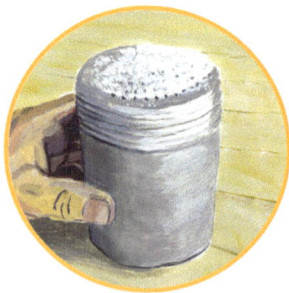

Then she almost dusted a little snow on her french toast. Kalea's family, who live in Hawaii, call powdered sugar "snow". In Honolulu, this is as close as they get to seeing snow fall, EVER!

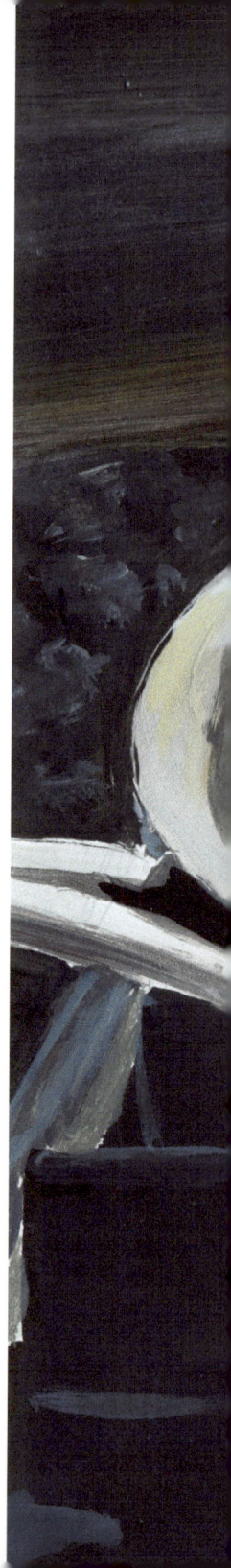

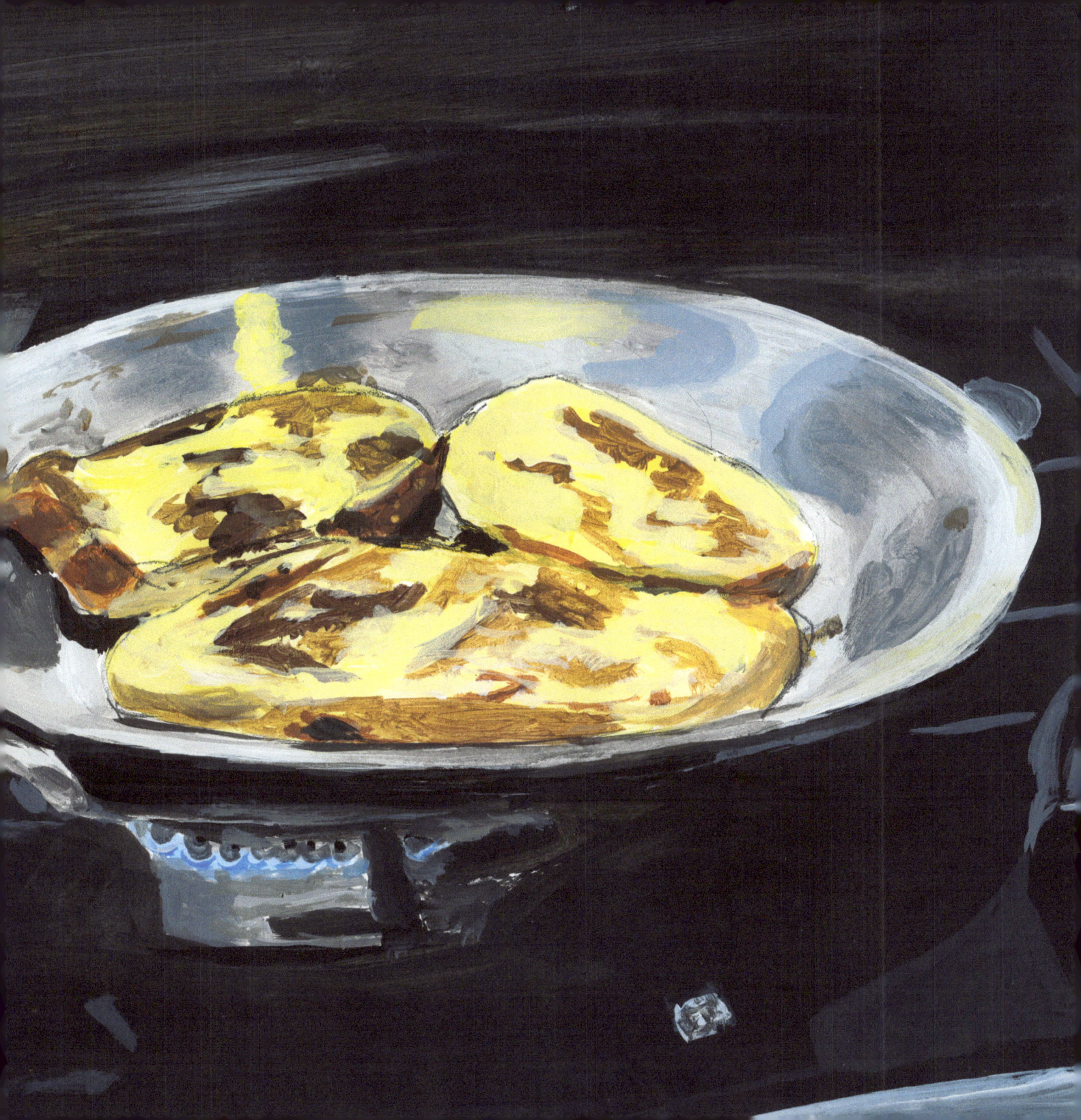

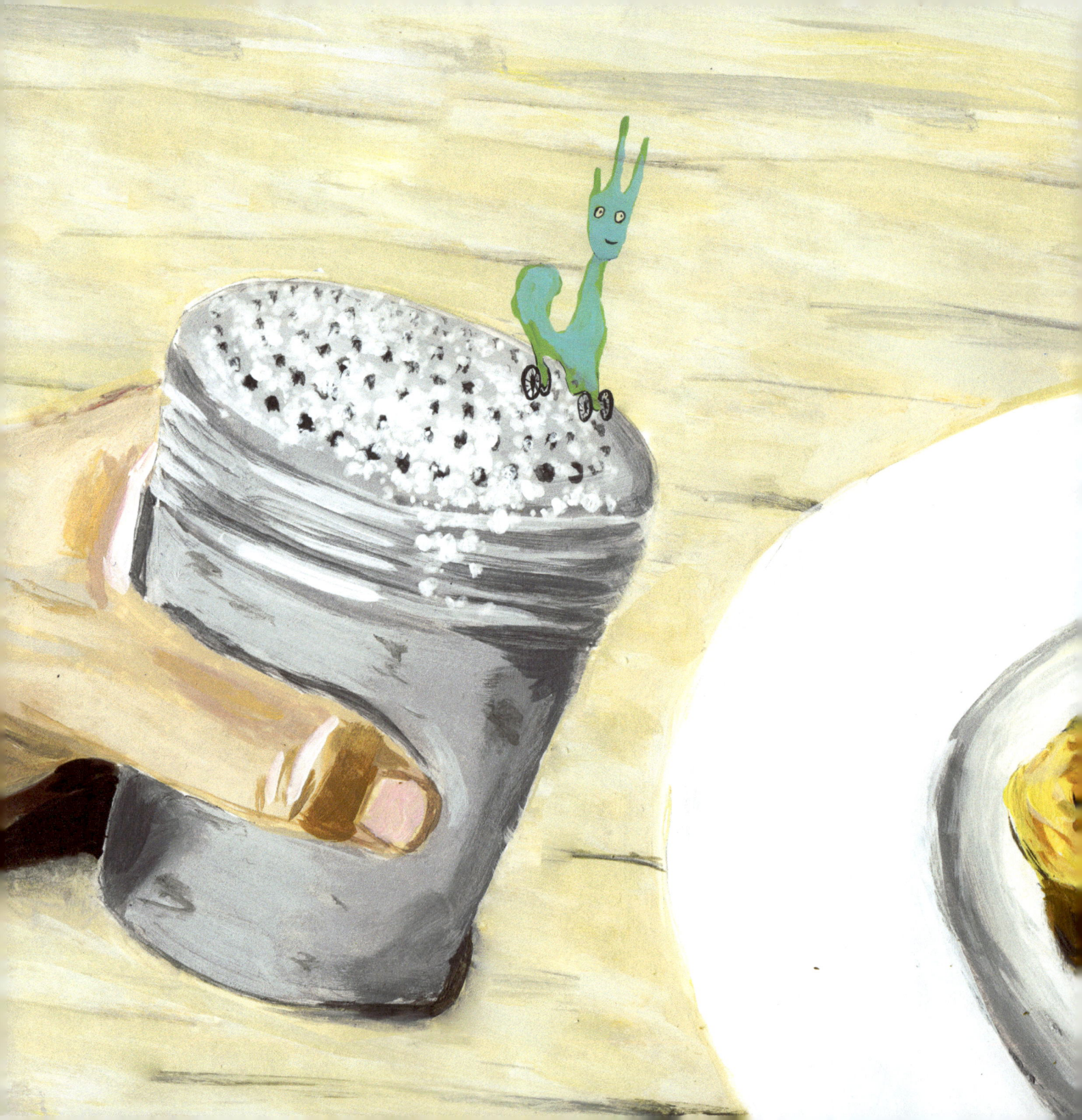

As she grabbed the duster, a strange little creature on wheels appeared.

"Oh, who are you?" Kalea whispered.

"Don't eat me. I am Sucrose, better known as Sugar: the Most Popular Sweetener in the World! I taste so YUMMY! I'm also known as granulated sugar, molasses, turbinado, muscovado, ...and ... evaporated cane syrup, demerera, powdered sugar, brown sugar, ..."

"Stop, I get it!" she cut Sucrose off. Kalea then proudly ate her plain french toast thinking about what to do next.

Day Two

The next day, Kalea went grocery shopping with her mom. She was so excited to search for food without sugar that she began singing to herself. "Cereal, cereal, boxes of cereal, which one has no sugar?"

"I'm here, I'm here, I'm here!" Sucrose said, rolling around everywhere.

"You again?" Kalea asked.

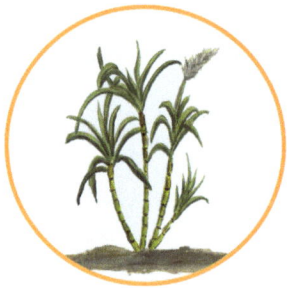

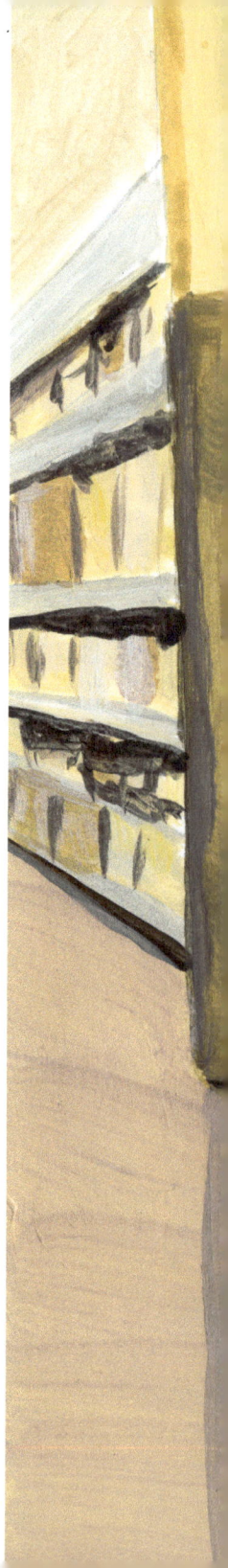

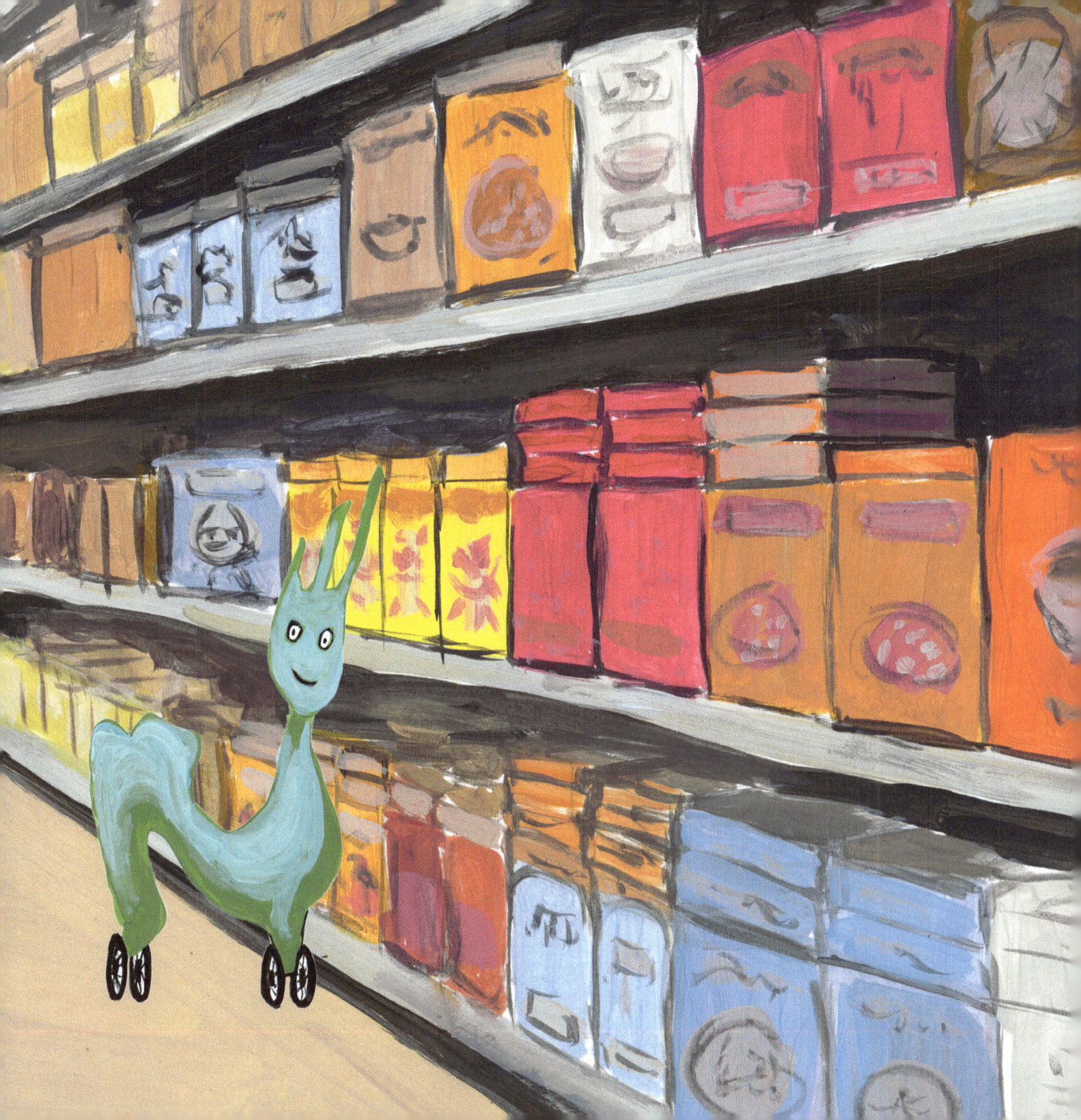

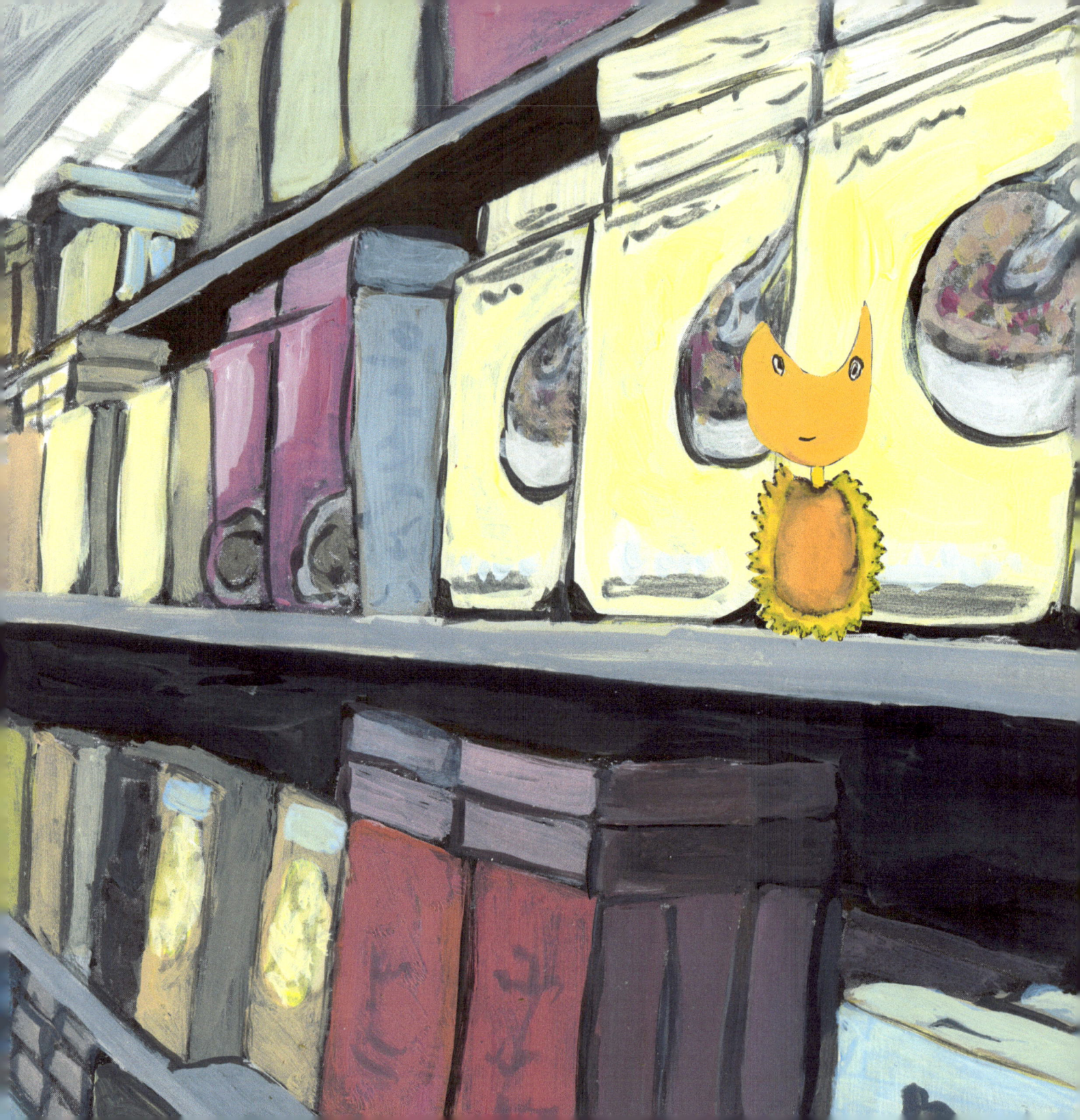

From behind a few granola cereal boxes, another little sweetener popped up.

"Hello, I'm Honey! Bees make me from flower nectar, and I've been used as a sweetener for 8,000 years."

"That's a long time," Kalea responded. "I learned from my gardening teacher, Miss Ami, that the bees are dying. Is that true?"

"Yes!" Honey exclaimed. "It's a huge problem. Humans are causing a lot of trouble for the bees and myself."

"I'm sorry, Kalea said. "Is there anything I can do to help?" But Honey was gone, so Kalea ran off to find her mom.

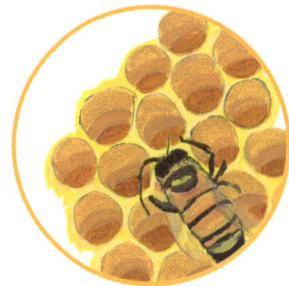

As Kalea passed the cookie aisle, she heard strange noises, like whispering kids playing hide and seek. She stopped and saw Sucrose, Honey and all kinds of other sweetener creatures scurrying away. One was even on a skateboard.

Later that day, a bored Kalea sat searching on the computer for a movie to watch. She found the documentary *Fed Up*, a movie about sugar.

As she watched the film, tears came to her eyes during the parts when they interviewed kids. The movie motivated her to continue her week without sugar and to see how it would make her body feel.

Kalea knew her brother, sister and parents had to watch the film. So, she convinced them.

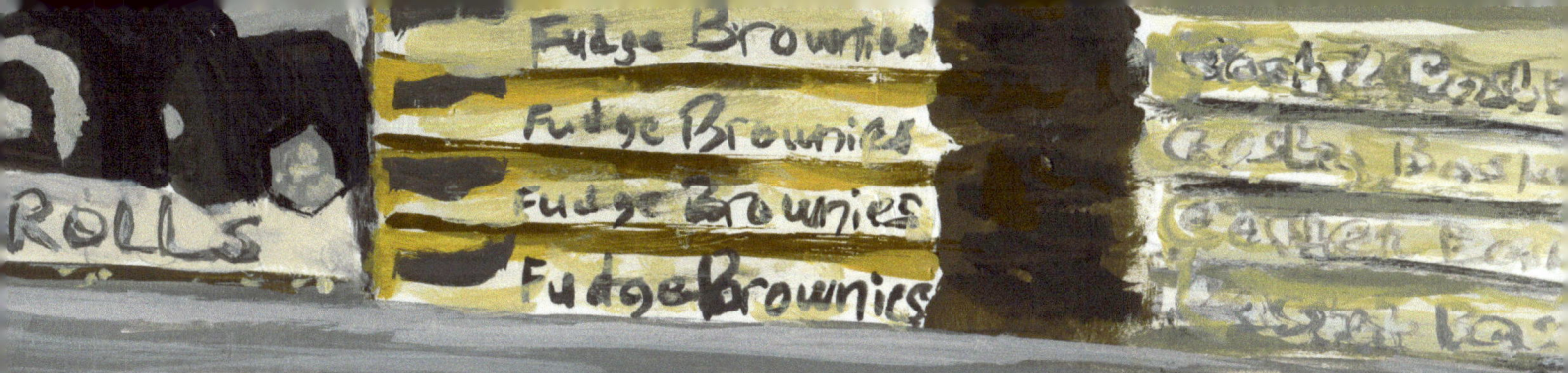

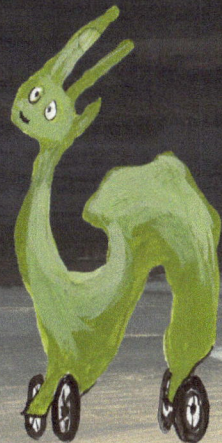

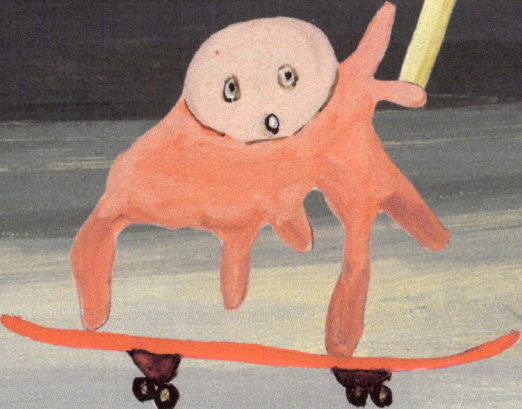

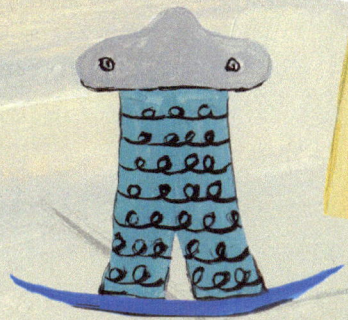

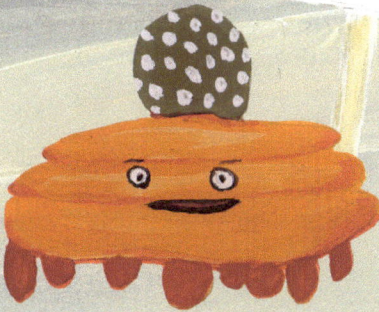

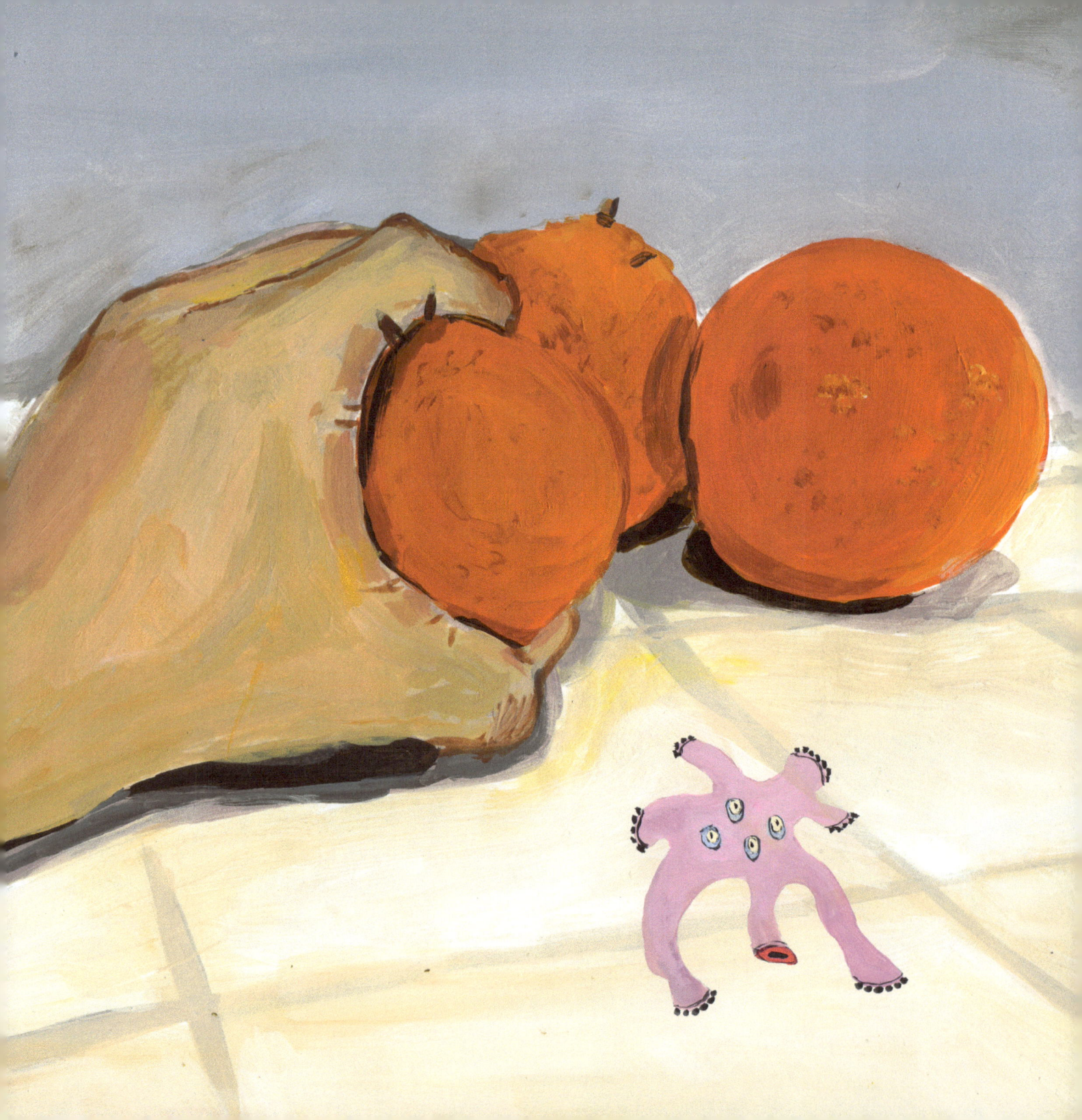

Day Three

The next morning, Kalea grabbed an orange, just when a strange creature erupted from the fruit. "Hello, I'm Fructose."

"Oh man, not another sweetener! Isn't fruit good for me?"

Fructose fluttered her eyelashes, "Yes, when you eat the whole fruit. But, if you see me listed as an ingredient, then I have been taken from a plant and made into a powder similar to sugar. It's not the same as eating a regular piece of fruit."

"Oh thanks, I guess I need to look for more than sugar on the ingredient lists," Kalea said.

"Keep up the good work!" Fructose said, as she squeezed back into the orange.

Day Four

After lunch at her grandma's house, Kalea snuck back into the kitchen to find some sugar-free cookies in the cupboard. Her grandma was diabetic and wasn't supposed to eat sugar.

"Who are you? The package says it's sugar-free." Kalea said feeling confused.

"I'm Sorbitol. That's Ace-K and Sucralose, my friends. We aren't sugar, we're sweeteners. I'm from the sugar alcohol family. I have less calories than sugar and I'm a little less sweet. I can be found in nature, but I'm made into a chemical substance from corn and other plants!"

"Hey, isn't that what happens to Fructose?" Kalea asked.

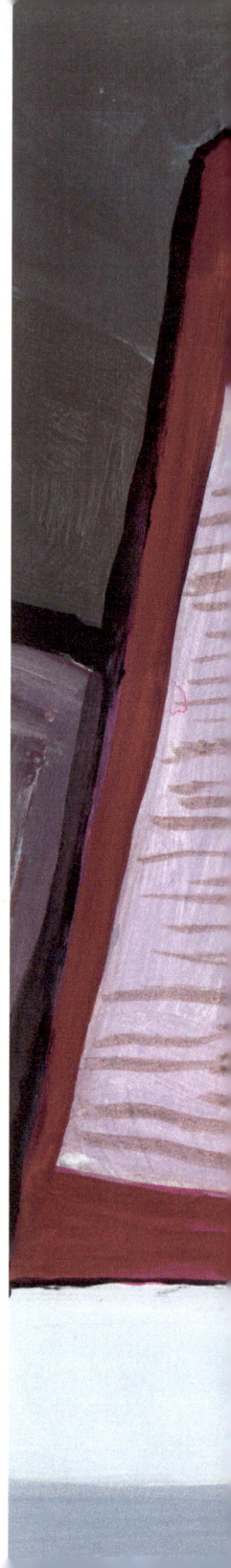

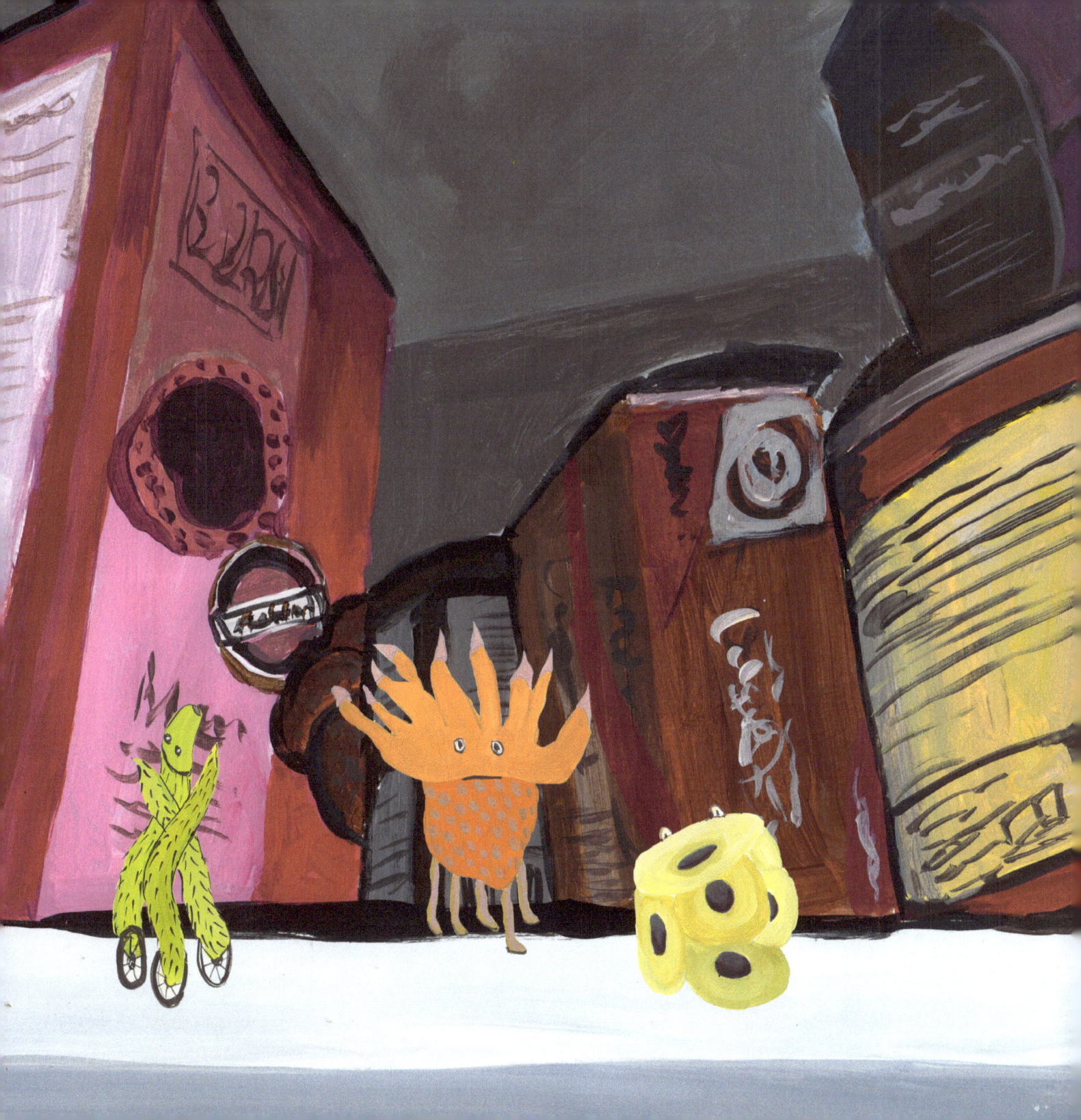

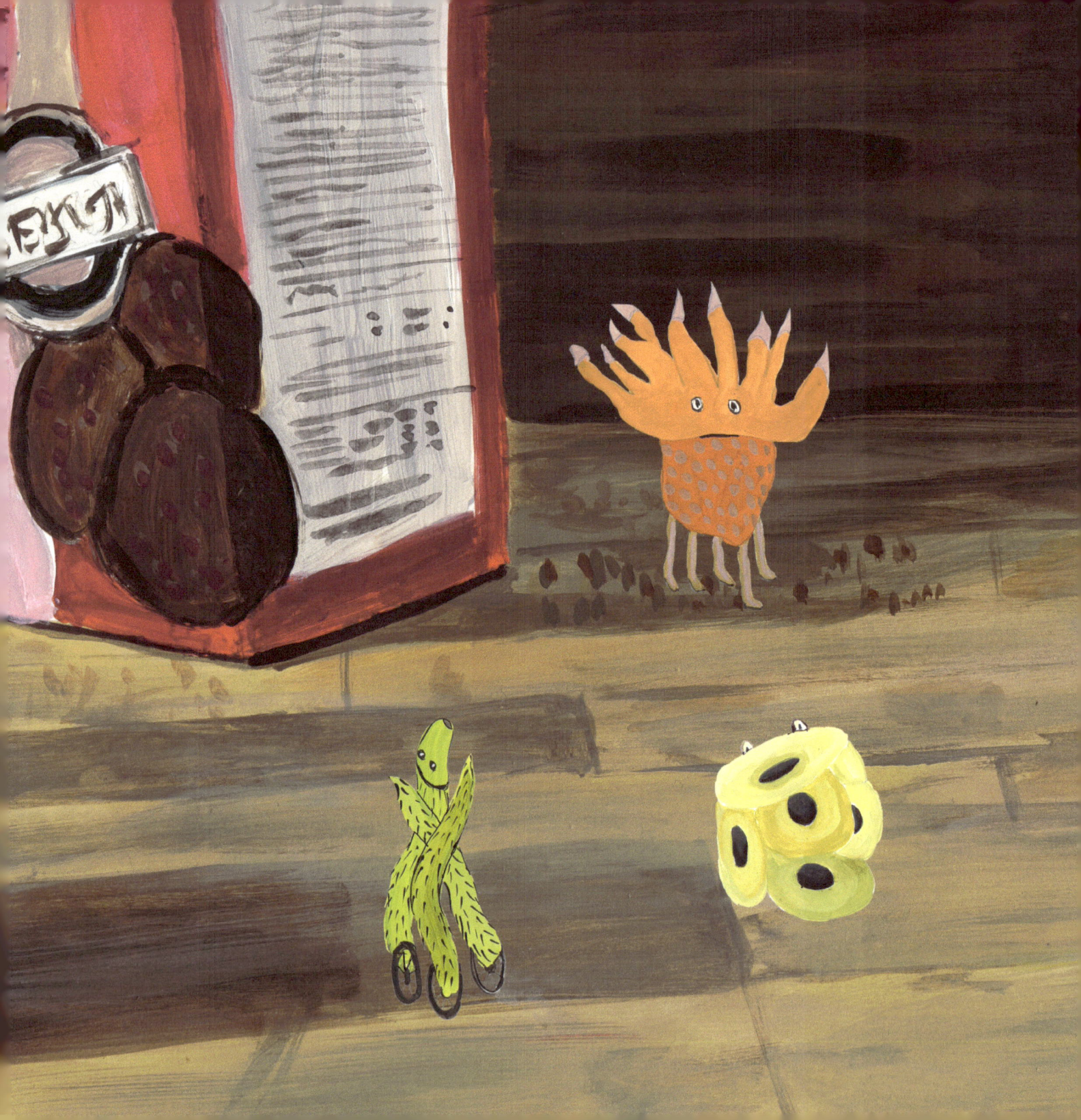

"Yeah," Sorbitol responded, "Kind of like Fructose, but I can give humans nasty stomach pain and bad gas if they eat too much." He snorted, "And they always do."

Sucralose said, "Ace-K and I are artificial sweeteners. Ace is 200 times sweeter than sugar and I'm 600 times sweeter!"

"Ace-K, that's a cool name!" Kalea marveled.

"My name's really Acesulfame Potassium, but we all got nicknames in the lab. Sucralose is also called Splenda."

Kalea slowly opened the package and ate one of the cookies. At first it tasted nice and sweet. After a couple of bites, she had this weird taste in her mouth. She grabbed some milk. "Oh, now I really want a homemade cookie!" she thought to herself.

After dinner, while Kalea was brushing her teeth, she thought about making it through four days of her sugar-free week. She was so excited until she looked in the mirror and saw something moving in her mouth.

"Hello, I'm Xylitol and I am a sugar alcohol from the birch tree."

She spit out the toothpaste, "What are you doing in my mouth?"

"I am often found in toothpaste and chewing gum since I help your teeth fight cavities," Xylitol said. "But, I also can poison dogs if they eat me."

"Oh, my freind Sammi has a cute little puppy. I'd better warn her about you," Kalea said, and then went off to bed.

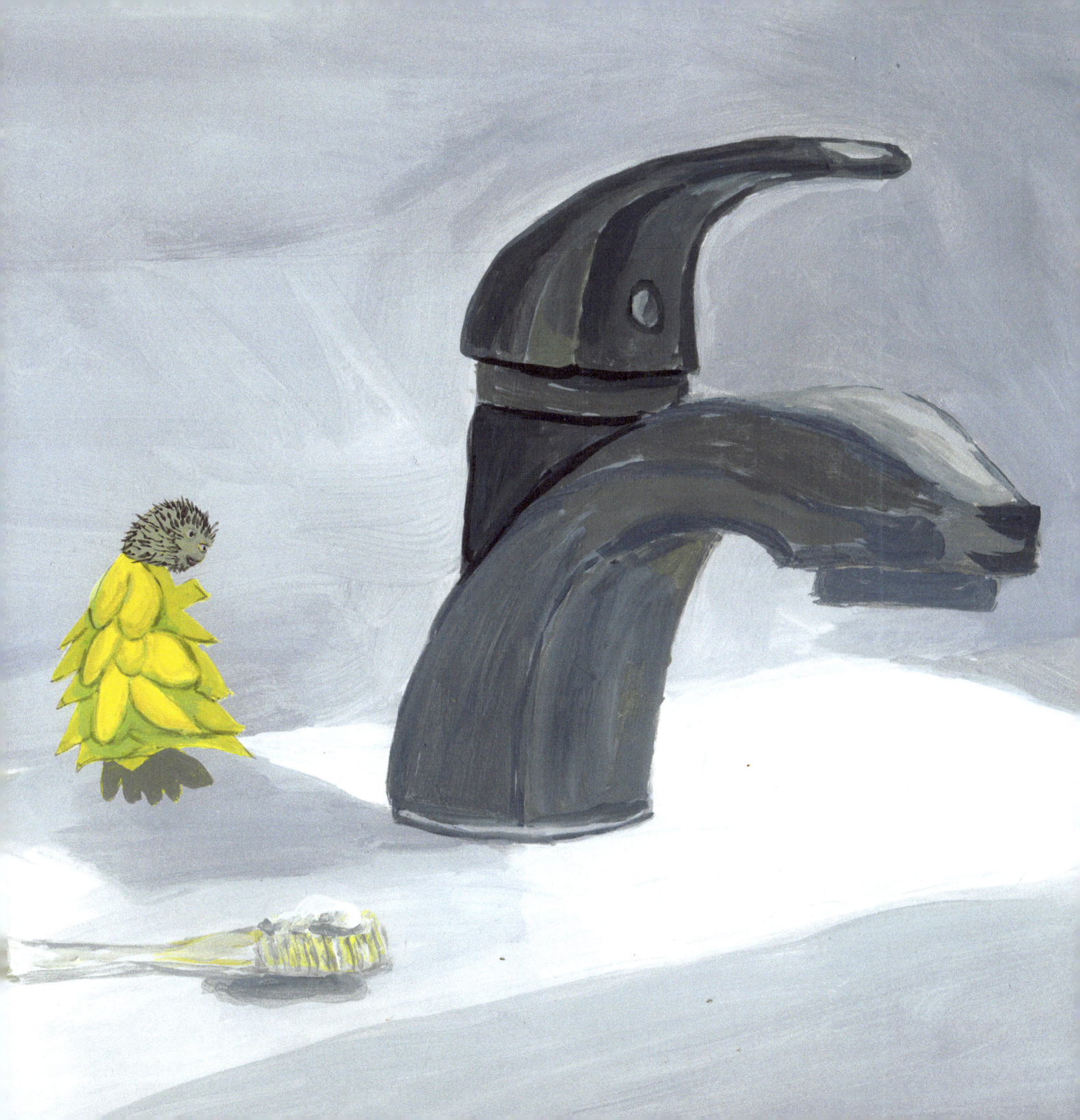

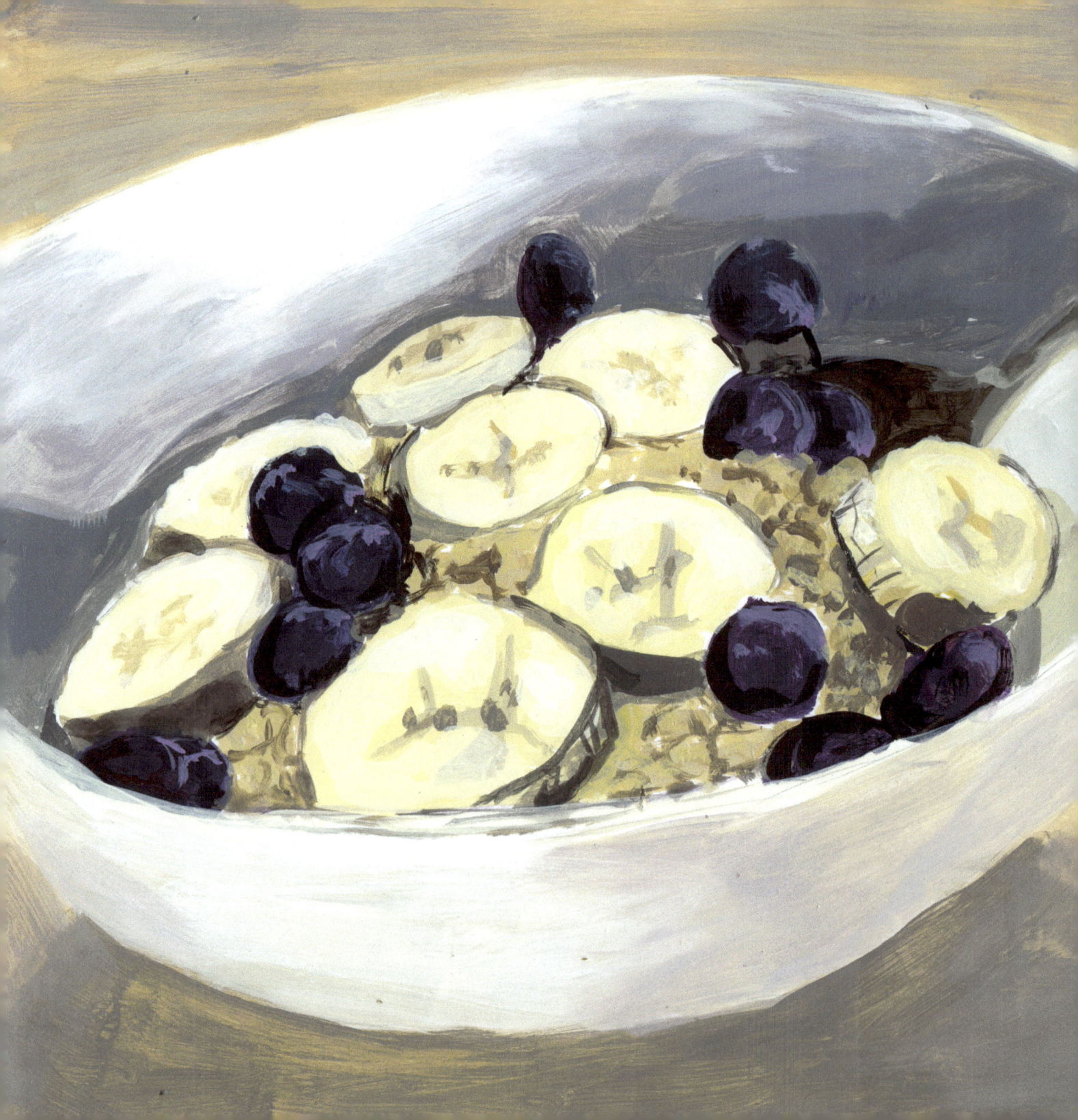

Day Five

Kalea was getting used to eating her oatmeal with bananas instead of brown sugar for breakfast. After surfing, she went to her friend Chenoa's house to play. Kalea recognized the lovely smell of chocolate chip cookies as she knocked on the front door.

"Oh cool, this is going to be such a fun day!" she said to Chenoa.

"But, I thought you gave up sugar for the week?" Chenoa asked, and then felt bad reminding her.

"Ohhhh Yeah," Kalea said. "They are my favorite! This is torture!" Then with a burst of strength, she said, "Let's go play soccer outside."

After playing soccer, Chenoa offered Kalea a stick of gum. When she opened the wrapper, she saw another creature. It was so small she barely saw it on the gum.

"Chenoa, do you see that guy? … Right there."

"Yeah, what is it?" Chenoa asked.

"Hey, I'm the reason the gum is so sweet. I'm Saccharin, the first artificial sweetener invented."

Chenoa dropped the gum on the floor. "That thing talks?"

"Dad," Chenoa hollered, "Why is there an artificial sweetener in my gum? You said we should only eat things with organic raw sugar, date sugar or something more natural."

"I guess I missed that," her dad said. "Want to try something really cool, … a miracle berry?"

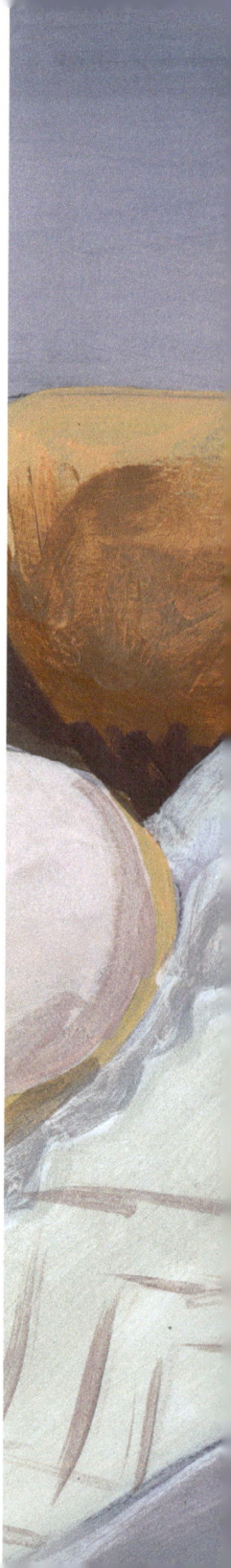

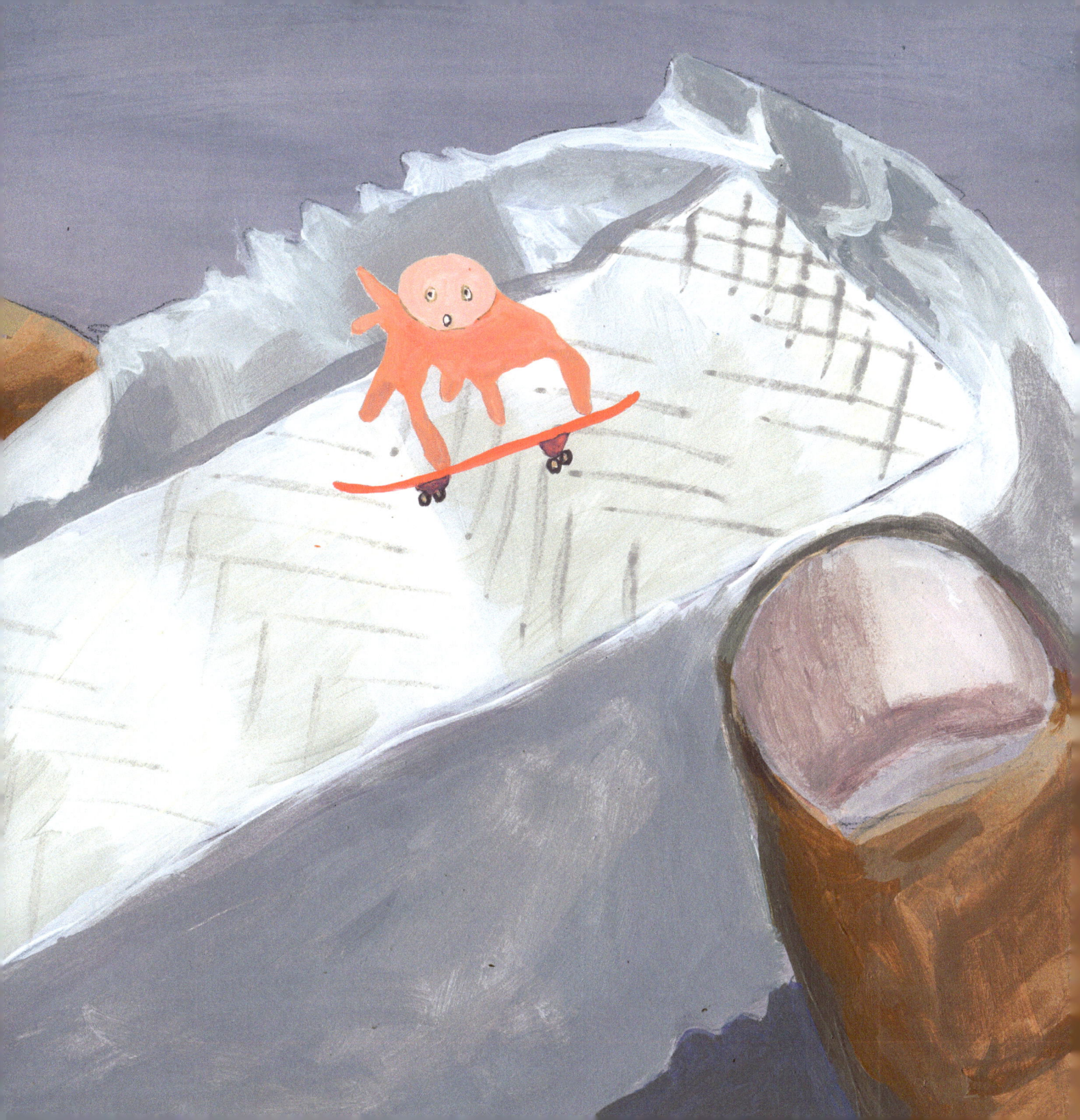

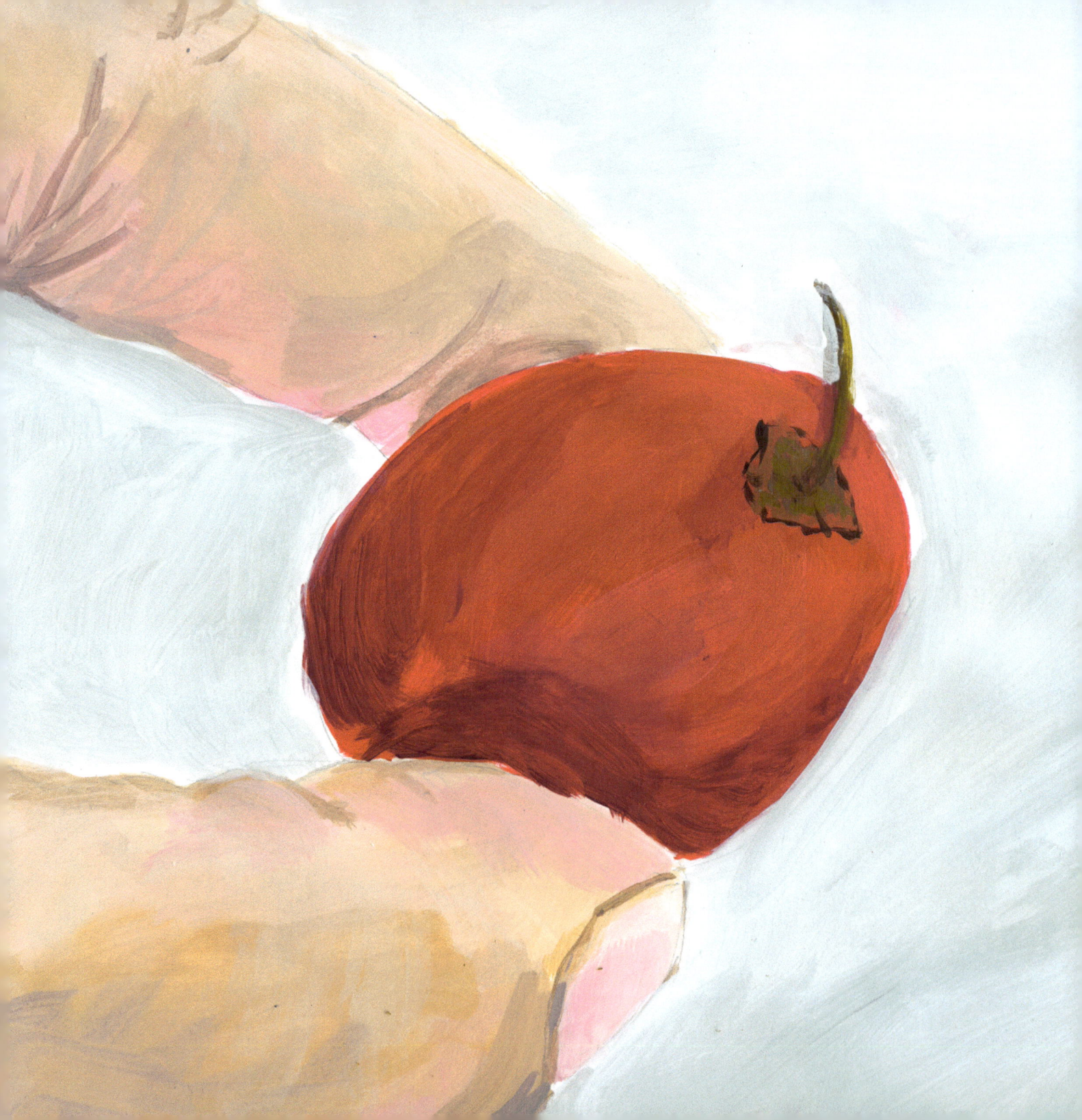

Kalea thought about it. "OK, I can eat a berry."
They each took a bite, but it didn't taste sweet at
all. It was kind of blah.

"Now try this lemon." Chenoa's dad cut them
each a slice with his chef knife.

"Ohhhh weird, it's sweet. That's really a lemon?"
Chenoa asked.

"Yeah, it's a lemon," Chenoa's dad said smiling.
"The miracle berry comes from West Africa. Some
people have used it for about three hundred years
to make bitter and sour food taste better."

They tried lots of things in
the kitchen over the next hour
until their taste buds went
back to normal. Kalea had such
a fun day, she forgot all about
the chocolate chip cookies!

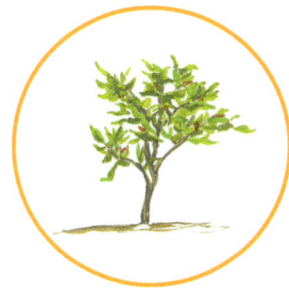

Day Six

Kalea spent the day at the beach reading a book and surfing with her sister. She was so distracted, she hardly thought about sugar at all.

That night, Kalea woke from her sleep in a sweat. She was in a laboratory similar to her mom's. She looked down at her white lab coat and saw hundreds of rats running around the corner toward her. She jumped up on the workbench and screamed.

They stared at her with sad, red eyes and began fidgeting nervously. Then they ran in circles around the lab bench. Just then, behind one of the chemicals next to her, another strange sweetener character crept out.

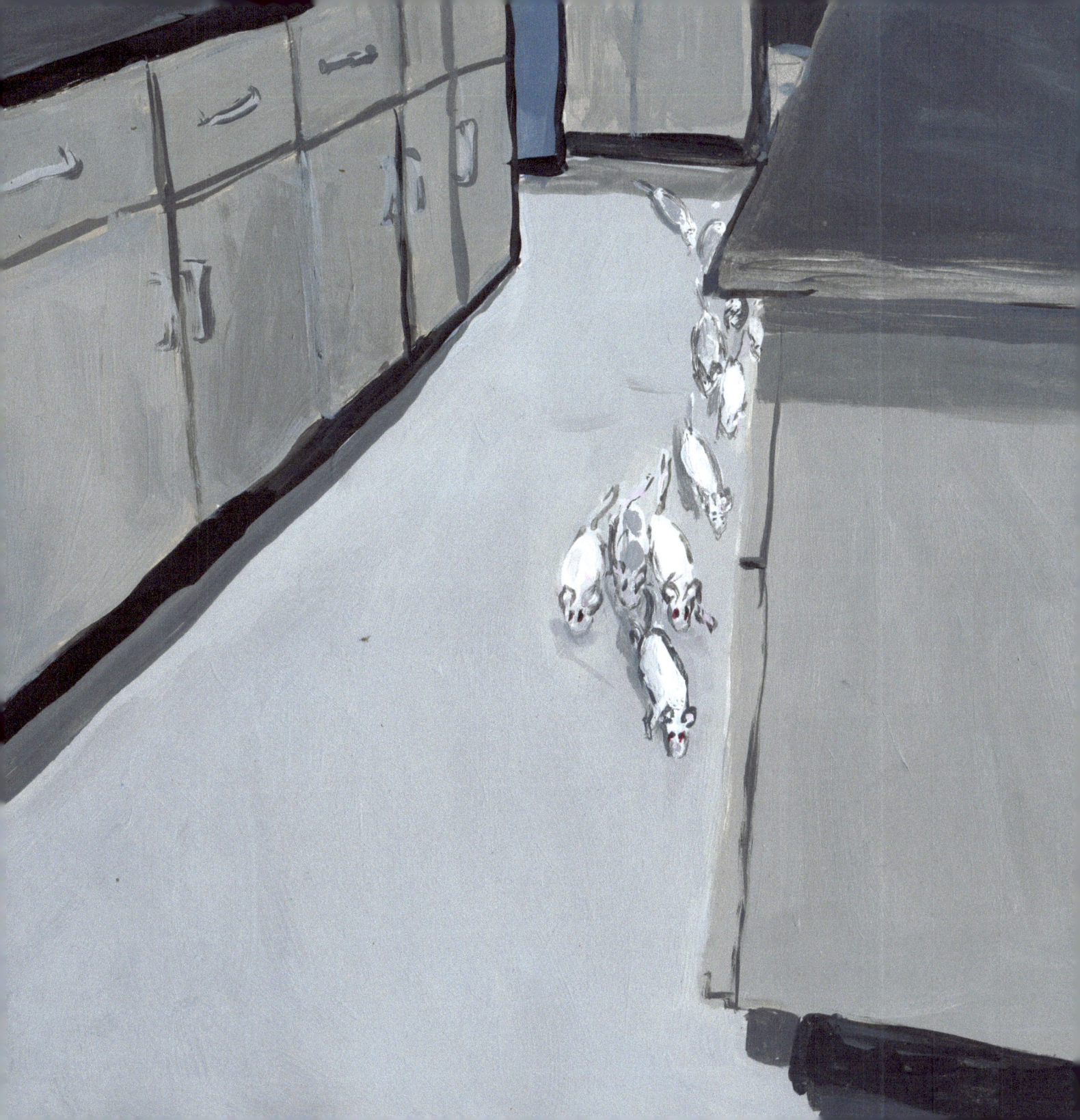

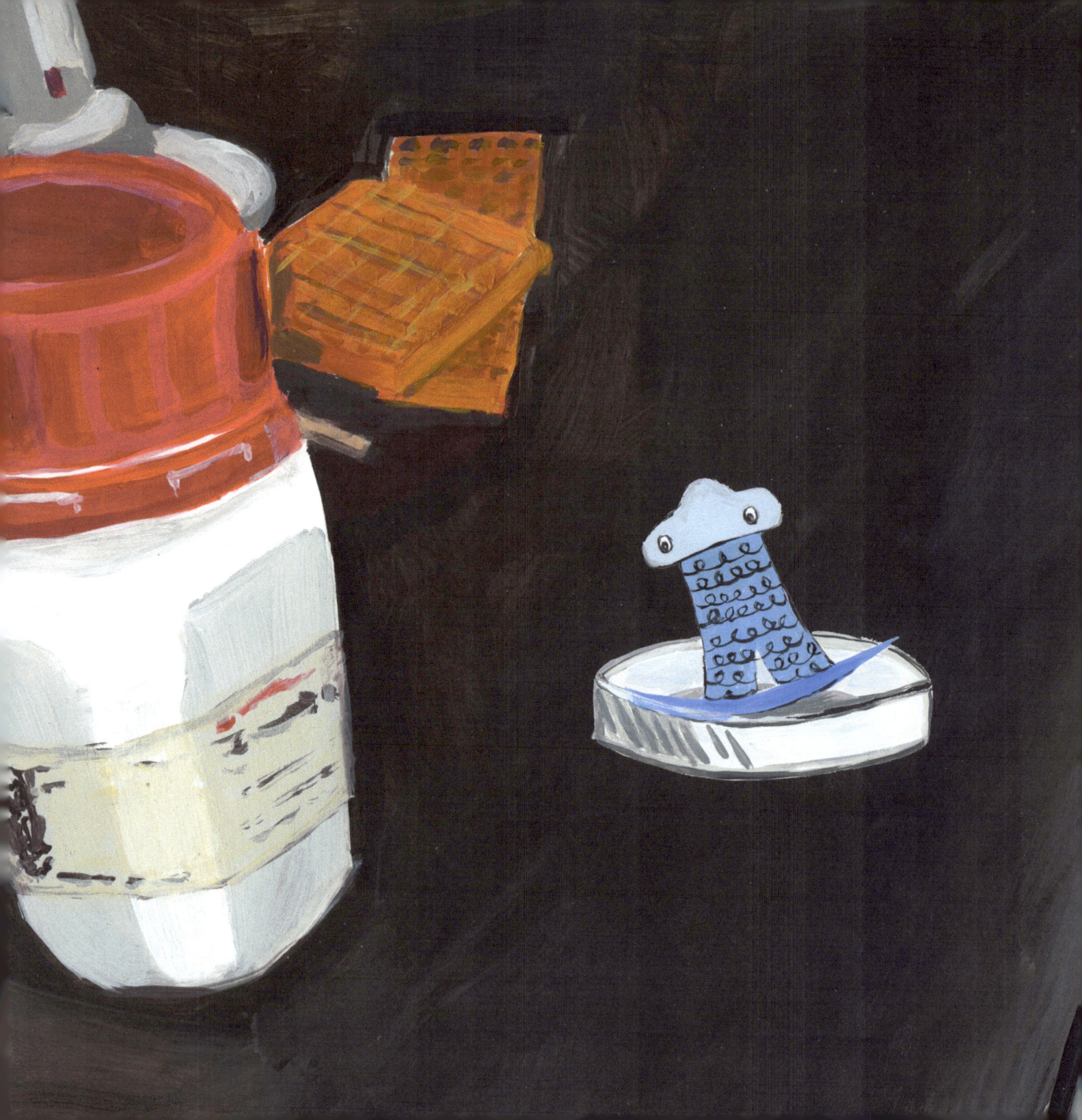

"Hello, I am Aspartame," the character snickered. One of the baby rats stopped, looked at Aspartame and cowered in fear.

"What are they running for?" Kalea asked Aspartame.

"I think they are tired of drinking me and are looking for some water."

Then, all of a sudden the rats were on the bench attacking Aspartame from all sides. That's when Kalea woke up feeling pretty freaked out. She'd never thought about all the rats used to test chemical sweeteners.

Kalea then drifted off to sleep dreaming about rescuing the rats.

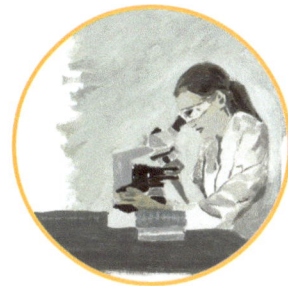

Day Seven

The following day she went to the school garden to help her mom pull weeds. On the way, she asked her mom, "What do you know about sweeteners?"

"Well," her mom said, "I think it's important to consider our health, but also the environment. It's pretty complicated, but I think it's better to choose organic and sweeteners that are least processed. Some of the artificial sweeteners that are up to 8,000 times sweeter than sugar might be okay because we use so little of them.

Scientists have also discovered that sweeteners like sucralose and ace-K survive through our waste stream after they leave our bodies and then end up in rivers and oceans. That might not be good for fish and plants further down the road."

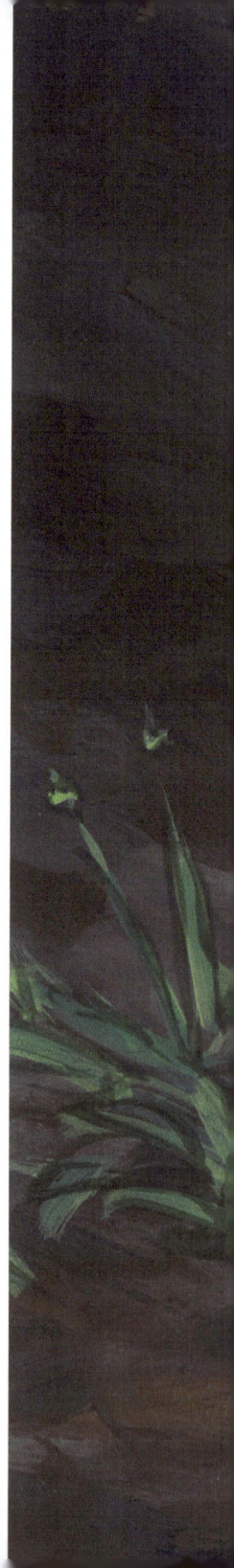

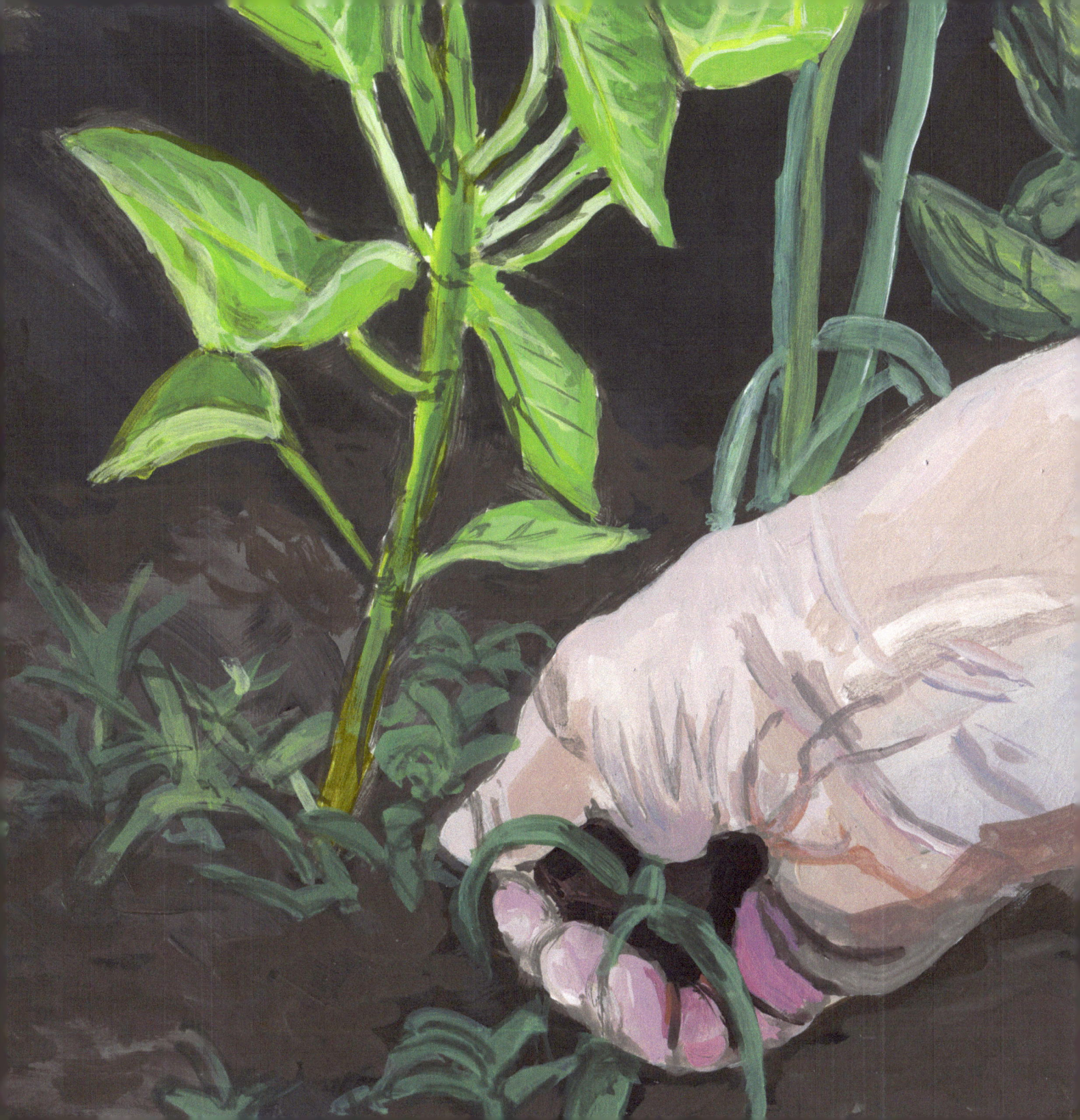

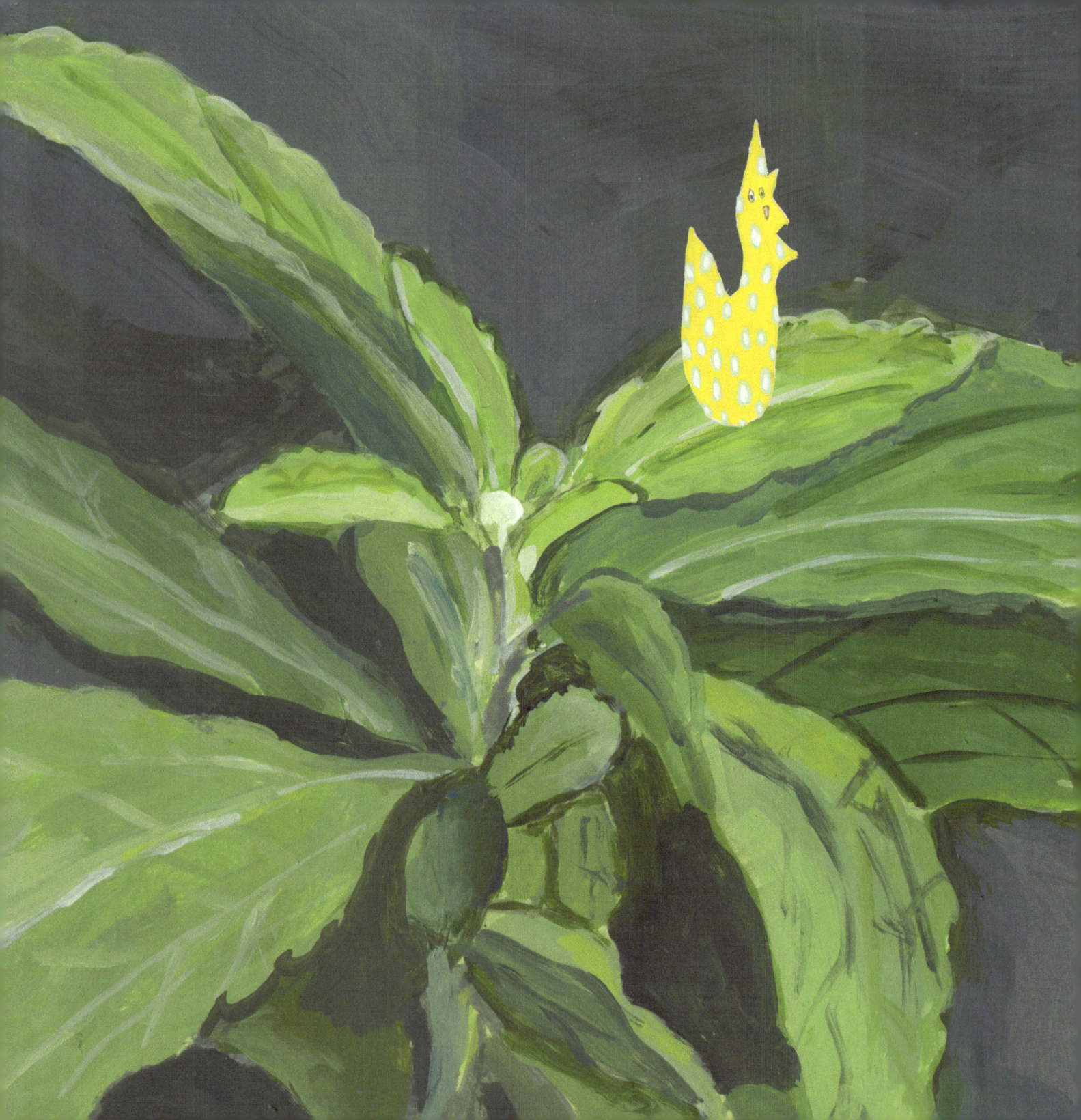

Again, the characters were popping up everywhere in the garden. Kalea recognized Fructose now. "Mom, is that tree called miracle berry?"

"Yes, we should have some ripe ones soon," her mom said.

"Who are you?" Kalea said to the little guy on the green leaf.

"Stevia is my name. Taste my leaf. I am also made into a white powder that is a lot sweeter than sugar."

"Wow," Kalea said. "That has a nice taste, a little like licorice."

"Yup, that's me! There's another sweetener like me with no calories that has been grown in China for centuries. It's also very sweet. It's called Lo Han Guo."

"Wow, Mom, can we plant some Lo Han Guo?"

That night Kalea slept at her cousin's house. "Evan," she said excitedly. "Guess what? This is my seventh day eating no sugar."

"Really,... well, I do that all the time." Evan said.

Evan's mom laughed as she poured him some cough medicine.

"Evan, do you see those guys?" Kalea asked.

"Where?" Evan said.

"They're jumping everywhere!" Kalea shouted. "See your spoon? They just jumped out of the bottle."

"Oh, wow, I see them now. What are they?"

"Those are all sweeteners in your medicine. Why are there so many?" Kalea asked.

"Because it's syrup," Evan giggled, as he drank it down quickly.

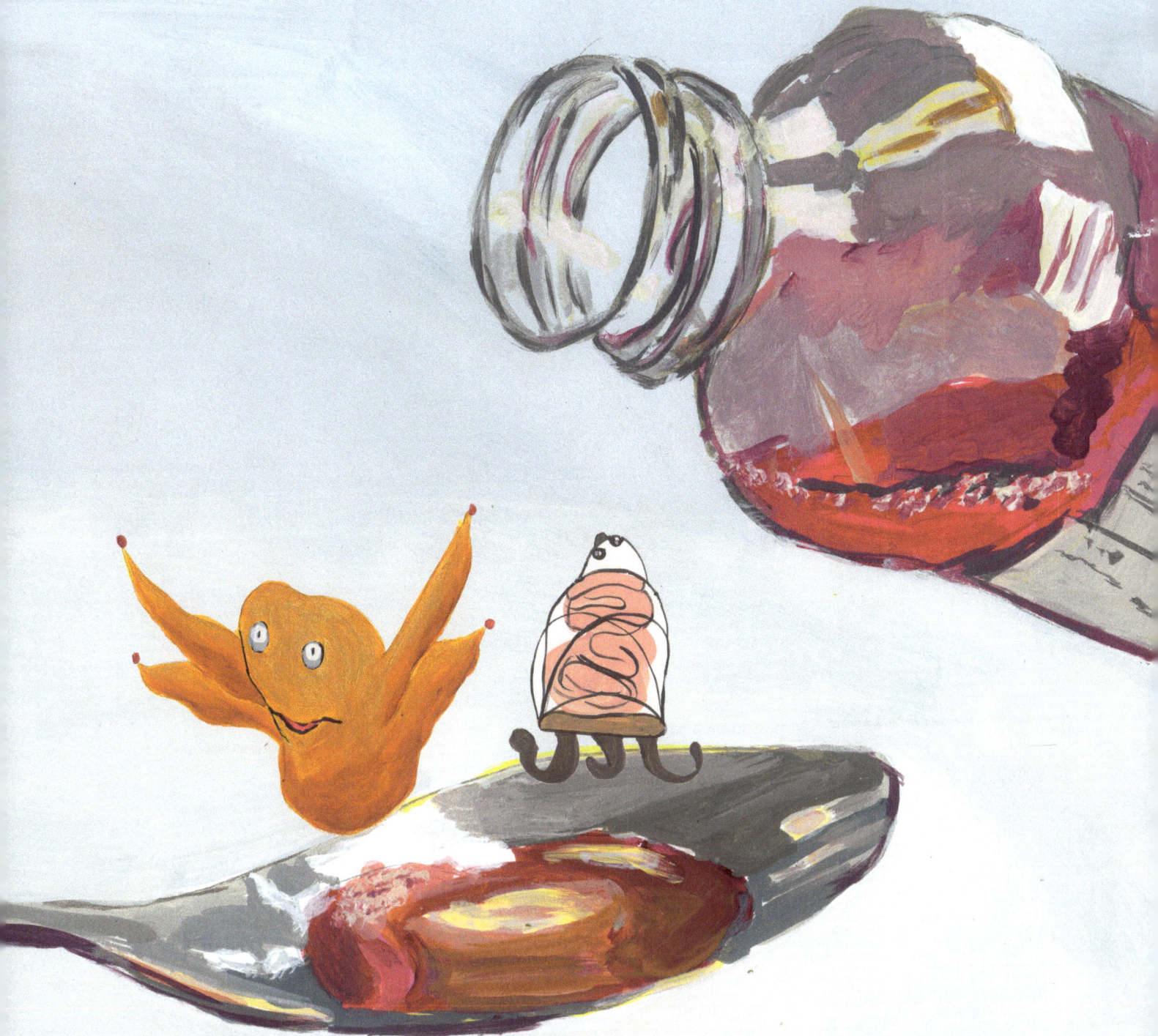

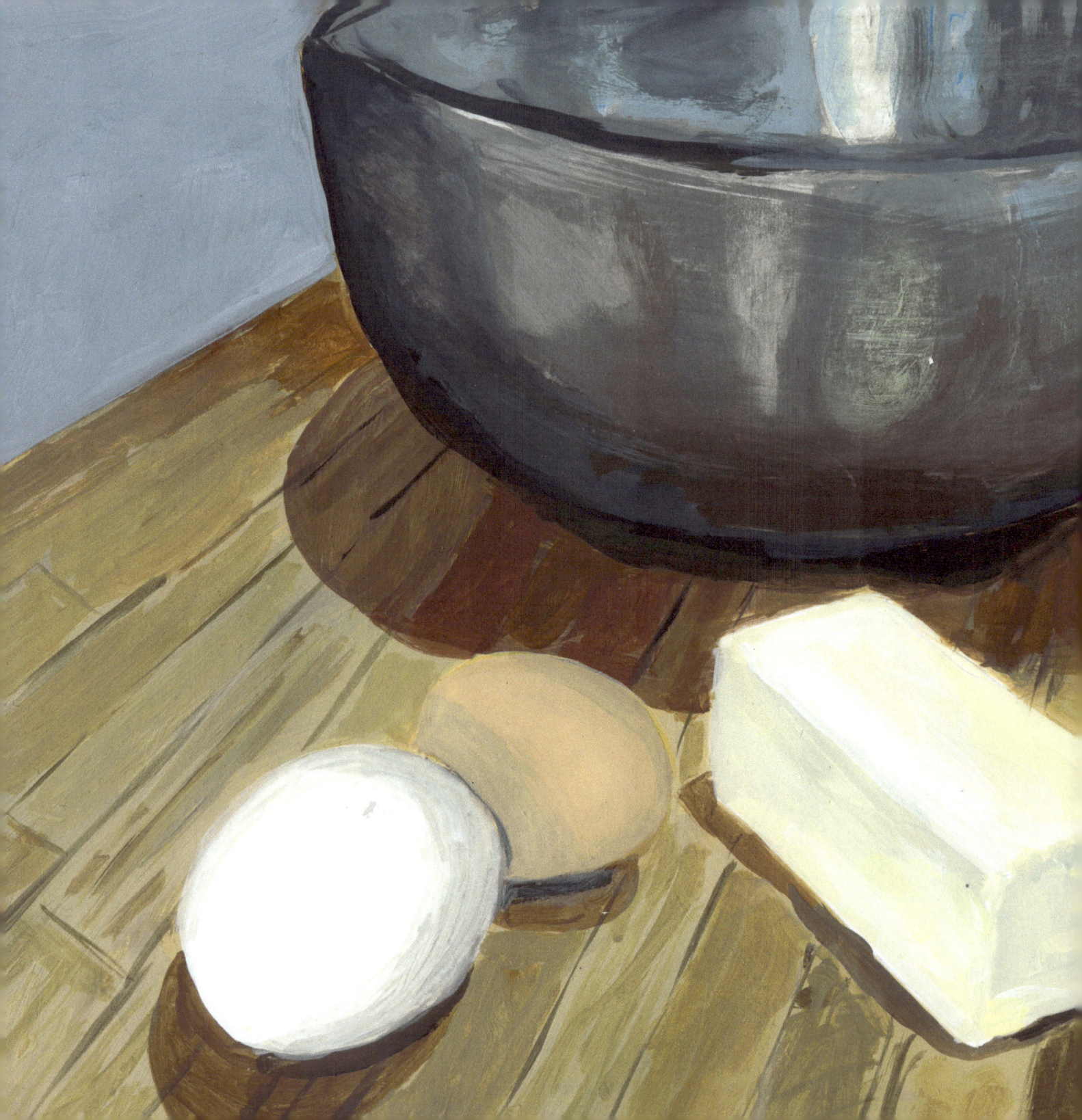

She Did It!

Kalea woke up early thinking about what she would eat to celebrate.

She yelled from her bed. "Mom, can you make me something sweet? I did my whole week without sugar. Can you believe it?"

"OK, I'll get up in a minute," Kalea's mom grumbled trying to fall back asleep. "I'm so proud of you, what do you want for breakfast? I think your cousin Ian is making breakfast for everyone this morning."

Kalea pondered about the past week. She learned a lot from the little sweeteners and hoped they would keep showing up.

Her garden teacher suggested she watch some short films that kids made near San Francisco called *The Bigger Picture*. She also couldn't wait to watch the documentary *More Than Honey* again with her friend Sammi.

Kalea enjoyed researching online about sweeteners. There, she found a new one that was 20,000 times sweeter than sugar. Kalea tried to imagine how that could be and whose job it was to taste them.

She was a bit torn about which sweeteners to choose, sugar alcohols, raw or less processed sugars, or super-sweet artificials.

Which would you choose?

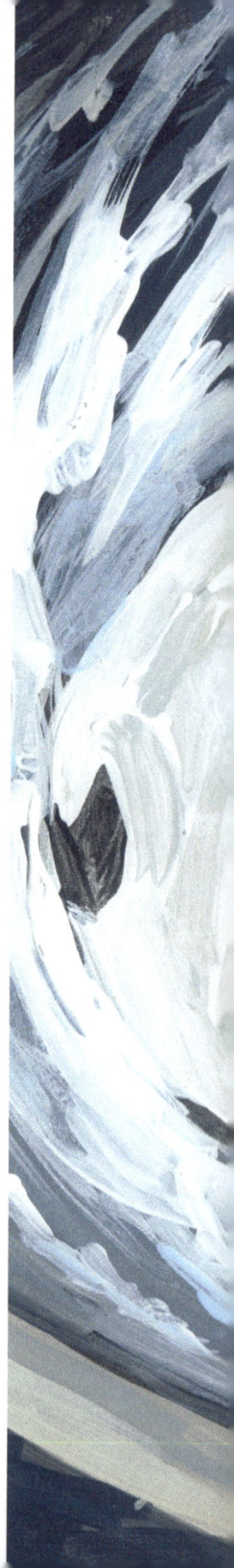

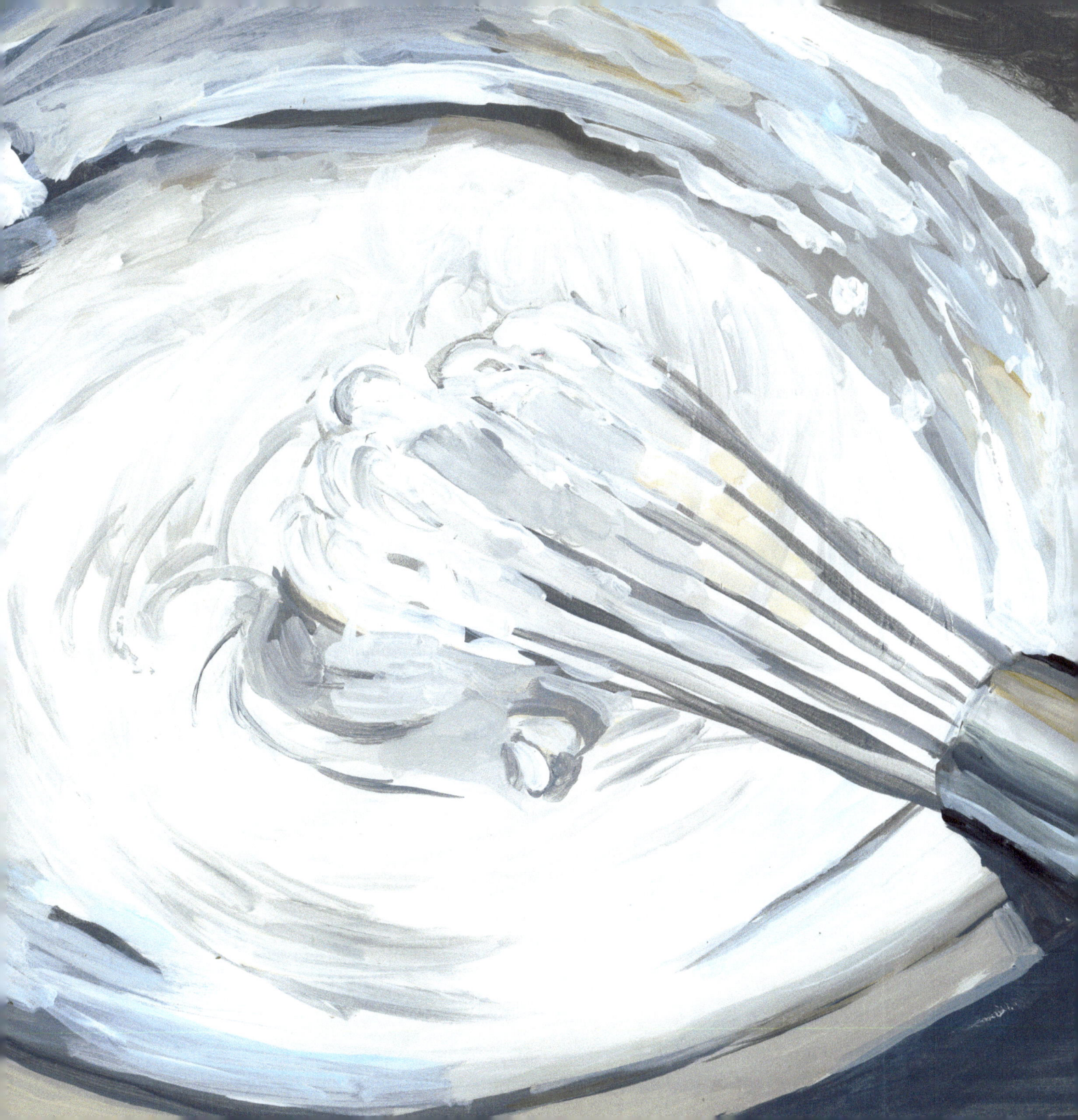

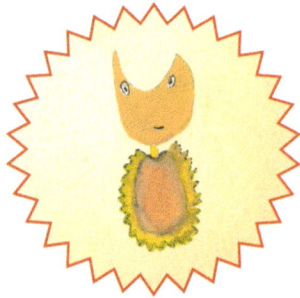

HONEY

- Has been used as a sweetener for 8000 years
- Is made by bees who collect and transform nectar
- Is also made by feeding bees high fructose corn syrup
- Can be eaten raw from a local farmer

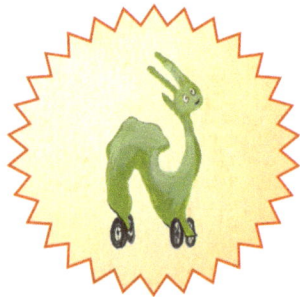

SUCROSE

- Comes from sugar cane and sugar beets
- Is minimally to highly processed in factories
- Can be made from organic or GMO crops

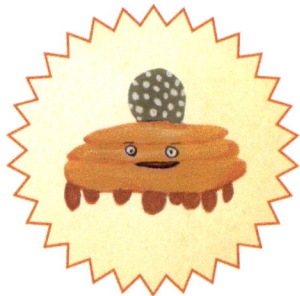

HIGH FRUCTOSE CORN SYRUP

- Comes from huge fields of GMO yellow dent #2 corn
- Is made in a factory and delivered in tanker trucks
- Is found in a lot of packaged foods and drinks

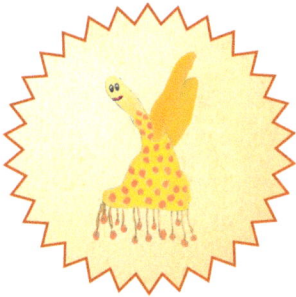

AGAVE NECTAR

- Was called by the Aztecs, "gift from the gods"
- Is made from the core of the Blue Agave plant
- Can be made from organic agave and less processed

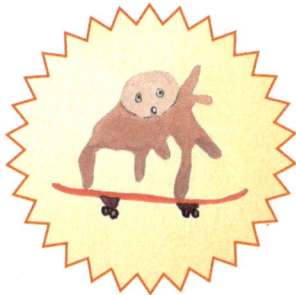

SACCHARIN

- Is an artificial sweetener first produced in 1878
- A.K.A. Sweet 'N Low
- Is 350 times sweeter than sugar
- Was discovered by a chemist licking his finger while working on coal tar derivatives

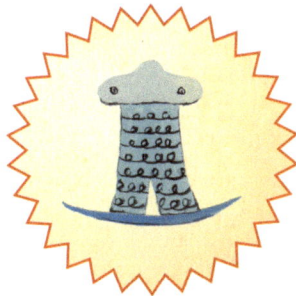

ASPARTAME

- Is an artificial sweetener A.K.A. Equal and NutraSweet
- Was discovered by a chemist licking his finger in the lab
- Is 200 times sweeter than sugar

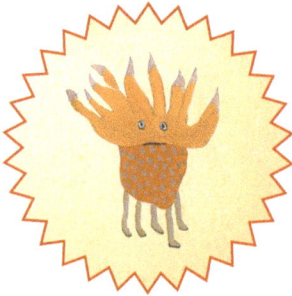

ACESULFAME K

- Is an artificial sweetener, A.K.A. Ace-K, produced in 1967

- Is 200 times sweeter than sugar and is found in beverages

- Was discovered by a German chemist licking his finger in the lab

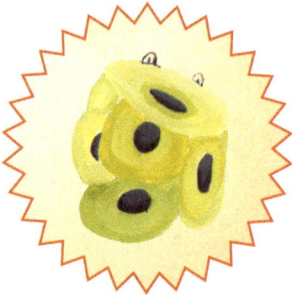

SUCRALOSE

- A.K.A Splenda, it is changed chemically from sucrose

- Was discovered in Great Britain when a graduate student was supposed to test it and instead tasted it

- Is 600 times sweeter than sugar

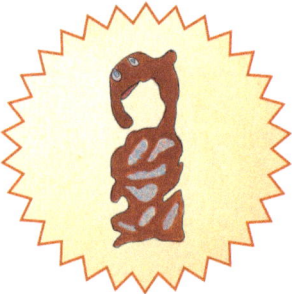

NEOTAME

- Is an artificial sweetener invented from aspartame

- Is usually added to beverages and foods

- Is 8000 times sweeter than sugar

- Newer Advantame is 20,000 sweeter than sugar

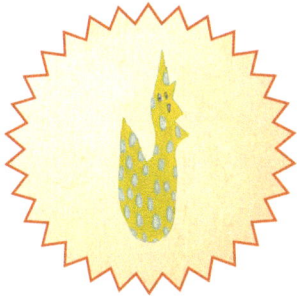

STEVIA

- Has been added to tea for 1500 years in S. America
- Can be eaten as a leaf or processed into a white powder
- Is made from the plant Stevia Rebaudiana, native to Paraguay

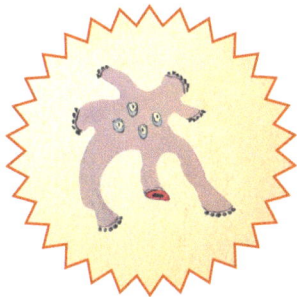

FRUCTOSE

- Is naturally found in honey, fruit, and root vegetables
- Has many names such as crystalline fructose
- Can be made into a powder from sugar cane, sugar beet or corn

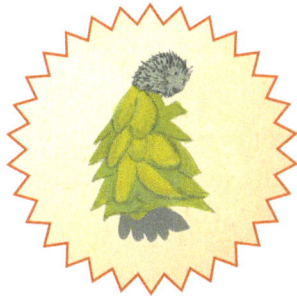

XYLITOL

- Is a sugar alcohol naturally found in some fruits
- Can be made into a powder from the birch tree
- Typically in gum, mints and toothpaste and can help prevent dental carries
- Is poisonous to dogs

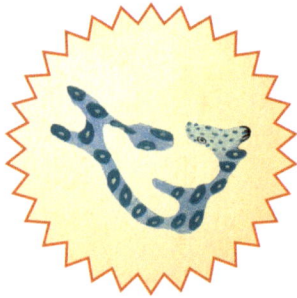

ERYTHRITOL

- Is considered one of the safer sugar alcohols

- Is often mixed with other sweeteners in products

- A sugar alcohol naturally found in some fruits and fermented foods

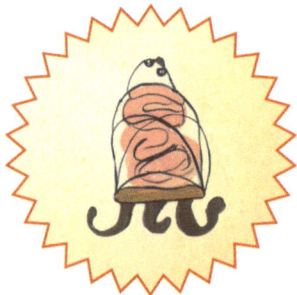

MALTITOL

- Is produced from the maltose in corn, potato or wheat starch

- Is a sugar alcohol with less calories than sugar

- Tastes a little less sweet than sugar

- Is used in baked goods, sweets and sugar-free products

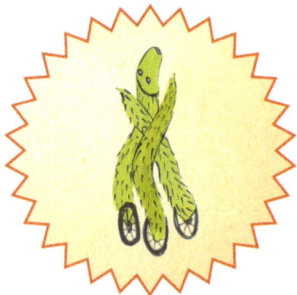

SORBITOL

- Is naturally found in fruit but is mostly processed from corn

- Sweetens like other sugar alcohols with less calories

- Is found in mints, diet foods, cough syrup and sugar-free chewing gum

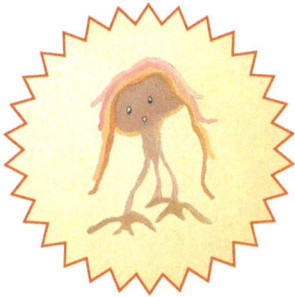

MIRACULIN

- Is made from a miracle berry into a powder
- Is a protein that has no calories
- Has a blah taste, but sour foods taste sweet for about
  an hour

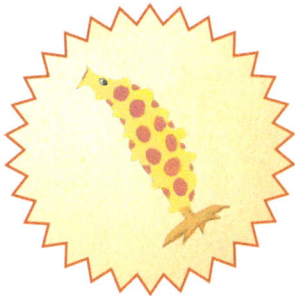

LO HAN GUO

- A.K.A. Monk Fruit Extract
- Was eaten as a whole fruit in the Tang dynasty by monks
- Created recently into a powder and not tested well
- Is 300 times sweeter than sugar

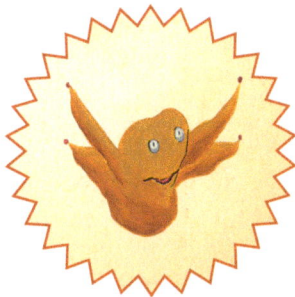

GLUCOSE

- A.K.A dextrose and grape sugar
- Is a simple sugar
- Is important for energy in plants and animals
- Is typically manufactured from cornstarch

BOOKS

Fat Chance: Beating the Odds Against Sugar, Processed Food, Obesity, and Disease by Robert H. Lustig (Dec 31, 2013)

Sugar Has 56 Names: A Shopper's Guide (A Penguin Special from Hudson Street Press) by Robert H. Lustig (Sep 3, 2013)

Sweet Nothings, Nutrition Action.com
The Center for Science in the Public Interest

FILMS

Fed Up, Stephanie Soeghtig, Director, 2014

More Than Honey, Markus Imhoof, Director, 2013

The Bigger Picture, Youth Speaks short films, Thebiggerpicture.org

www.ingramcontent.com/pod-product-compliance
Lightning Source LLC
Chambersburg PA
CBHW060856270326
41934CB00003B/165